ESSENTIAL OILS FOR BEGINNERS

THE LITTLE KNOWN SECRETS TO ESSENTIAL OILS AND AROMATHERAPY FOR WEIGHT LOSS, BEAUTY AND HEALING

Ella Marie

© 2015 Sender Publishing

Table of Contents

INTRODUCTION

You might have heard another celebrity raving about their new beauty product, a rare oil from Morocco, or maybe you have witnessed the transformation of a friend's skin from dry and lackluster to stunningly supple and radiant. When you question your friend about the magical elixir that brought about this rapid change in the quality of her skin, she utters "essential oils." Your interest is now piqued; you are revved up and ready to discover the world of essential oils, and you plan to use them daily to affect positive changes throughout your life. Yet a couple of keystrokes later, you find that discovering the realm of essential oils will not be such an easy task after all. The search term 'essential oil' yields 47,300,000 results on Google and each page has its own bit of information with its own fact and fiction. If only you could find a book that presents information about essential oils with the facts to back it up – a book that gives the practical uses of essential oils and recipes that you could use to create even more potent oils by mixing two or more existing oils.

This is your eureka moment, for you have found the book that will do all that and more. In this book, I will introduce you to the topic of essential oils and aromatherapy. I will give comprehensive information about essential oils and their origins, properties, uses, storage, and safe use. By the time you finish this book, you will be well equipped with knowledge of how to determine the quality of essential oils in terms of their purity, grade, and integrity.

So, read on if you are ready to take that step to becoming an essential oil connoisseur; I promise you, it's a decision you will not regret.

CHAPTER 1
WHAT ARE ESSENTIAL OILS?

Essential oils are not a new fad that has popped up in the last couple of weeks; they have been around for ages and have been used by people worldwide for cosmetic, spiritual, medicinal, and emotionally uplifting purposes. Essential oils are the natural aromatic compounds extracted from the barks, seeds, roots, stems, flowers, and other parts of plants. The term "essential oil" is derived from the original term 'quintessential oil' from ancient Aristotelian ideas. Aristotle believed that matter was made up of five elements: air, fire, water, earth, and the fifth element, or the 'quintessence,' thought to be the spirit or life force of the matter. Hence, essential oils are thought to contain the characteristic fragrance of the plant along with all of its beneficial properties.

Nowadays, we know that there is no such element known as the "quintessence," but that does not mean that essential oils do not exist. They do exist, and they play important biological roles in the plants that manufacture them. Most essential oils attract pollinators to their plants by the alluring scents that they give off. This is biologically important for plants since they need to be pollinated by insects and small animals to survive, but we humans have found these scents to be soothing and sometimes invigorating too. Essential oils also play the role of defense in plants because of their antibacterial and antifungal properties; they play the same antibacterial and antifungal roles when applied to our skin and have even been shown to stimulate the regrowth of healthier and stronger skin. So, you see, essential oils have important alluring, protective, and regenerative properties that we can make use of if we know how to utilize them properly.

In fact, essential oils have been used by different civilizations and different cultures for thousands of years. Read on and discover how ancient civilizations extracted and used different essential oils from different plants and how you can use them today.

CHAPTER 2
HISTORY OF ESSENTIAL OILS

EGYPT

Evidence indicates that the ancient Egyptians were using aromatic oils as early as 4500 BCE. They were an important part of the Egyptian culture because they were used for religion, cosmetics, meditation, healing, and other aspects of life.

The Ancient Egyptians concocted a famous herb mixture made of sixteen different and specially-blended ingredients to create a substance known as "Kyphi." Kyphi was used as a perfume, as a medicine, and also as incense.

Special essential oils were allocated to each Egyptian god and even pharaohs were given their own unique blends. At one point in Ancient Egyptian history, only the priests were allowed to have certain essential oils because those essential oils were deemed necessary for intercessions with their gods.

CHINA

The Chinese first started using essential oils between 2697 and 2597 BCE; this was during the reign of the legendary Yellow Emperor, Huang Ti. It is believed he authored the booked called "The Yellow Emperor's Book of Internal Medicine." This book contains a vast amount of information about several essential oils and aromatics, and it is still utilized by many Eastern Medicinal Practitioners today.

INDIA

Traditional Indian medicine known as the "Ayurveda" has been utilizing essential oils in healing potions for over three thousand years. Their medicinal scripts list over seven hundred substances (such as ginger, cinnamon, sandalwood, and myrrh) and their essential oils as potent healers. It's interesting to note that Ayurvedic medicine was successfully used to replace the ineffective antibiotics that were present during the outbreak of the Bubonic Plague. In addition to their medicinal purposes, essential oils were also used philosophically and spiritually by Ayurvedic practitioners because they were believed to be a godly part of nature.

GREECE

The Greeks adopted the knowledge of essential oils from the Egyptians and recorded them between 400 and 500

BCE. They also adopted the knowledge of Ayurvedic medicine from the Indians and incorporated it into their existing body of knowledge.

It was this mixture of knowledge from Ancient Egypt and Ancient India that the Greek physician Hypocrites, also known as The Father of Medicine, used to document the effects of some three hundred different plants, including saffron, thyme, cumin, marjoram, and peppermint. Hippocrates has made an important contribution to modern medicine as we know it today, and all doctors have to take a pledge, known as the "Hippocratic Oath," in honor of the late Hippocrates.

Another notable Greek, who put plants and the essential oils that they contain to good medicinal use, was Galen. He was a surgeon at a school for gladiators, and it is said that no gladiator who was placed under his care succumbed to his injuries and died. Galen made good use of essential oils, and soon he was promoted to being the personal physician of the great Roman emperor Marcus Aurelius. Galen did extensive research on plants and their properties and divided plants into many different medicinal categories. Some of these categories are even used to this day.

Greek soldiers also made use of essential oils. They carried ointments of Myrrh with them to treat infections when they went to battle.

ROME

The Romans made use of essential oils in different ways. Instead of using them medicinally, they used them for cosmetic and therapeutic purposes, and they were known for the huge quantities of perfumed oils that they applied to their clothing, bedding, and bodies. It was also customary for Romans to use essential oils in their baths and in massages.

Roman physicians were avid readers of the literature produced by Hypocrites and Galen, and during the fall of the Roman Empire, the Roman physicians fled to other lands with copies of these ancient texts. These texts were later translated into different languages, such as Arabic and Persian.

PERSIA

A child prodigy known as Ali-ibn Sana (also known as Avicenna the Arab) became a popular and erudite physician by the tender age of 12. He wrote several books about eight hundred plants and their different effects on the human body. He was also the first person to discover and record the method of distilling essential oils from plant materials. His methods of distillation are still used today.

EUROPE

The knights and their armies passed on extensive knowledge of herbal medicines that they learned throughout Western Europe and the Middle East during the time of the Crusades. The knights acquired the knowledge of how to distill the essential oils from other civilizations, and they used them to make perfumes.

In the 14th century, during the time of the Bubonic Plague, the Europeans burned pine and Frankincense in the streets to ward off "evil spirits." Fewer people actually died from the plague in the areas where this was done.

Many Europeans came up with valuable literature that is still used in some areas today. Chief among them were the French chemist René-Maurice Gattefossé and Nicholas Culpeper.

It was René-Maurice Gattefossé who coined the term "aromatherapie" while he was investigating the antiseptic properties of essential oils, and he later went on to publish a book in 1928, which vividly describes essential oils and their healing properties. This book had a profound influence on the medicinal practices in France at the time. René-Maurice Gattefossé discovered the healing properties of lavender because of an accident that had occurred in his laboratory in which he was badly burned. To lessen the pain of the burn, he quickly immersed the affected hand in the liquid that was closest to him. This liquid was the essential oil of lavender, and to his surprise, the wound healed with no scarring or infection. After this discovery, he, along with some other colleagues, conducted extensive research on the healing properties of lavender, and soon lavender was being used in all the hospitals across France. When the Spanish influenza eventually made its way to the country of France, no hospital personnel died as a result of illness, and this was credited to their extensive use of lavender and other antiseptic essential oils.

"The Complete Herbal" is a book that contains valuable reference material about many different medical conditions and their remedies using the essential oils of plants. It was written by Nicholas Culpeper in 1653, and it is still used today.

So, you see, essential oils have been used for several different purposes since the dawn of time. "But how did they remove the essence from the plants?" you may ask. Well, this was done in several different ways.

CHAPTER 3
HOW ARE ESSENTIAL OILS MADE?

You may be surprised to know that main method used to make essential oils has been around for more than five thousand years. This method is distillation, and it works by slowly forcing water or steam up through the plant materials to remove the volatile components. These volatile components (which consist mainly of water and the essential oil) are then cooled, and then the essential oil is separated from the water.

Another method that is used that is similar to distillation is percolation or hydro-diffusion. The difference with this method is that steam is forced through the plant materials from the top instead of the bottom.

There is another method used in essential oil extraction that is worthy of discussion. This method is used to extract mainly citrus essential oils, and it is called expression. In this method, no heat is involved, but instead the oil is forced from the plant material via mechanical pressure.

You may wonder what would be the difference between an expressed essential oil and its distilled counterpart. Well, expressed oils are considered to be more stable than their distilled counterparts, and they usually have a better aroma. Nonetheless, you can use any of the essential oils and reap the benefits from them as long as they are suitable for your use. But how would you know a suitable essential oil from a fake one – how could you tell the quality of an essential oil? Read on into the next section; your answers await you.

CHAPTER 4
DETERMINING THE QUALITY OF ESSENTIAL OILS

So many factors can come into play and affect the overall quality of an essential oil. Anything that affects the plants from which you extract the essential oil will affect the final quality of the oil. Therefore, environmental temperature, soil quality, and growing conditions play a major part in the overall quality of the final product. The techniques that you use to extract the oil can also affect the quality of the essential oil. If you can remember from above, it was noted that expressed oils had a better quality than their distilled counterparts, and this was due only to the method used to extract the oil. Despite all the different factors that can come into play and affect the quality of the essential oil, there are three main things that you the buyer should look for: grade, integrity, and purity.

GRADE

You should not use the grade as the only method for determining the quality of an essential oil because, like everything else, grading is subjective, and one person may consider a particular sample to be of a mediocre grade while another person considers it to be normal. Grading is often done just to determine which essential oil is best for a particular use. Yet the grade of a particular essential oil will give an indication as to its quality, so it should not be completely ignored when you are purchasing your essential oil. Always ensure that you buy an essential oil that was extracted for therapeutic use and is of a high grade.

INTEGRITY

Integrity here simply refers to whether or not an essential oil is from a natural plant source, as opposed to being manufactured in a laboratory or chemically altered. Essential oils with integrity do not separate (which would indicate that they have been diluted with some kind of vegetable oil) when they are frozen, and they do not have an alcoholic odor (which would indicate that some alcohol was placed in it).

PURITY

A pure oil is one which has not been diluted in some way. Some manufacturers like to dilute the essential oils that they sell with alcohols, vegetable oils, similar smelling essential oils, and other solvents so that they can use less of the real essential oil and make a profit at the same time. Always test for the integrity of the essential oil before you buy it.

CHAPTER 5
ESSENTIAL OILS: SAFETY AND STORAGE

If you've just bought yourself a bottle of a coveted essential oil, you may be thinking of ways that you can store it and keep it safe so that it can last for a long time. Follow these tips and tricks and your essential oils will be with you for years to come.

Always store your essential oils in dark-colored bottles away from direct sunlight. The dark-colored bottles will filter out the ultra-violet light which would otherwise cause the essential oils to break down. In the past, they were always stored in amber-colored bottles, but even dark blue bottles are fine.

The bottle should be kept tightly closed in a cool location. It is important that the temperature of the essential oil does not vary much throughout the day because this too can cause it to break down. You may refrigerate it, but that is not necessary.

You should also keep essential oils out of the reach of animals and children. Animals and children are very curious and they may open or break the bottles, ingest the contents, or cut themselves. As such, you should ensure that you keep your essential oils out of their reach.

It is also important that you do not store your essential oils in areas where there are sparks or flames. Many essential oils such as peppermint, pine, orange, and fir are highly flammable, so err on the side of caution and keep your essential oils away from open flames and sparks.

CHAPTER 6
POPULAR ESSENTIAL OILS

LAVENDER OIL

Lavender is one of the most popular essential oils you will find on the market, and this is because of its different health benefits. It is known to relieve pain, eliminate nervous tension, enhance blood circulation, treat respiratory problems, disinfect the skin, and scalp among other things.

Lavender oil is made from the flowers of the lavender plant, Lavandula angustifolia, which primarily grew along Mediterranean coasts. It then slowly spread to the rest of the world as more people became aware of its usefulness and versatility. The lavender oil is extracted primarily through steam distillation. These flowers are fragrant by nature and have traditionally been used for the making of potpourri. Interestingly, it takes about one hundred and fifty pounds of lavender leaves to produce only one pound of lavender oil, and, on average, an acre of land will only yield about twelve pounds of lavender oil.

You're probably used to seeing lavender as an ingredient in different perfumes, lotions, gels, infusions, soaps, aromatherapy oils, and ointments, and I am sure you will be surprised when you discover that there is a world of other benefits that lavender bestows on those who utilize it. It also blends well with many other essential oils, including pine, cedar wood, geranium, nutmeg, and clary sage.

COMMON USES OF LAVENDER OIL TODAY

Bug Repellent: Most bugs, such as midges, moths, and mosquitoes, cannot tolerate the potent smell of lavender essential oil, so you can use it when you go outdoors for an effective, sweet-smelling bug repellent. Simply apply a few drops of the lavender oil to the parts of your skin that will be exposed when you are outside and those pesky critters will avoid you.

Lavender oil is also anti-inflammatory, so if one of those annoying critters does get to bite you, simply apply a few drops of the lavender oil to the affected area and say goodbye to the swelling and the pain.

Sleep: If you're having trouble sleeping at night, lavender can step in and help. Did you know that it has been used to induce sleep in insomniacs for ages? Yes, it has! Lavender oil has a calming effect on the nervous system, and it has been proven to increase sleep regularity in people who apply a few drops of it to their pillow before they retire for the night. In fact, it has had such a calming and sleep-inducing effect on some people that those people have been able to use it to completely replace the sedatives that their doctors prescribed for them to sleep better at night.

Nervous system: Lavender oil's calming effect on the nervous system makes it an excellent tonic for anxiety and for the nerves. The refreshing aroma increases mental activity while at the same time removes nervous exhaustion. You can use it to combat your headaches and migraines, and you can also use it to relieve emotional stress, nervous tension, and depression. A study was conducted in which some students, who were about to take a test, were asked to inhale some rosemary and lavender oil. You'll be happy to know that the test takers who inhaled the rosemary and lavender oil showed significant decreases in anxiety and other forms of mental stress. There was also an increase in their cognitive function, so use lavender oil regularly and with confidence, knowing that it is good for your mind.

Acne: If you listen to the advice of notable aromatherapists and dermatologists, lavender essential oil will be one of the main substances you utilize in your fight against acne. They say that it is one of the most powerful substances that can be used to treat acne in both teenagers and adults alike.

Acne is a condition that occurs when there is a build-up of sebum near the sebaceous glands because of a bacterial infection. The bacteria feed off of this sebum and later proliferate. As a result, the area gets infected, then it gets irritated and then visible sores can be seen, sometimes with some amount of scarring.

Yet lavender oil has been proven to work wonders on acne-afflicted skin because it not only inhibits bacterial growth, but it also promotes blood flow to the affected area and thereby encourages healthy skin cell formation. It also reduces the over-production of sebum, and this helps to reduce and prevent acne formation.

To make use of this powerful anti-acne essential oil, simply put a few drops of it on a swab of cotton and then apply it to the affected area. You may have to alter this procedure to fit your individual needs because if your skin is sensitive, it would be more advisable to dilute the lavender oil before you apply it to your skin. It will still have the same properties, just in a milder form.

Lavender has also been used to treat many other skin disorders such as psoriasis, wrinkles, other inflammatory conditions, and even scar tissue. Lavender oil speeds up the healing process of cuts, wounds, burns, and sunburns. So feel free to use lavender oil to improve the overall quality of your skin.

Pain Relief: Lavender oil is excellent for relieving different types of pain, even those caused by rheumatism, sore and tense muscles, sprains, muscular aches, lumbago, and backache. Joint pain can also be relieved by using lavender oil to massage the affected area. Say bye-bye to your aches and pains forever when you choose to use this potent pain reliever.

Respiratory Disorders: Lavender oil is also widely used in the treatment of various respiratory problems, including colds, coughs, the flu, bronchitis, whooping cough, sinus congestion, tonsillitis, and even laryngitis. Its stimulating nature helps to loosen and eliminate phlegm that blocks the respiratory surfaces and causes congestion. The antibacterial properties of lavender essential oil and its vapor also help to fight off respiratory tract infections. To relieve respiratory disorders, apply the lavender to the skin of your back, chest and neck, or you can add it to your inhaler or vaporizer and inhale the vapor.

Hair Care: Lavender oil has been shown to be very effective against lice eggs, lice, and nits. Those insects won't want to be neighbors with the lavender oil and will quickly evacuate their home (your scalp) when you rub it daily with a few drops of lavender oil. Lavender oil has also been shown to be very helpful in the treatment of hair loss, especially in people who suffer from Alopecia, a condition in which the body rejects its own hair follicles, and it is also effective in the fight against male pattern baldness. Simply rub the lavender oil into your scalp and watch the difference.

Blood circulation: Having poor circulation? Lavender oil is the way to go! It improves blood circulation to the organs of the body and thereby increases their levels of oxygenation. It promotes muscle strength and even boosts brain activity. When you use lavender oil regularly, your skin looks brighter and healthier because it is constantly being flushed with blood. It also lowers blood pressure and protects you from arteriosclerosis and heart attacks, which are diseases often associated with poor circulation. Even diabetics who often suffer from low circulation can make use of this product by applying it to the affected areas or inhaling the vapor from an inhaler or vaporizer.

It is important to note that you should not combine lavender with sedative drugs. You can use it to replace the drugs, but do not combine them because doing so will induce too much sleepiness.

CLARY SAGE OIL

You have probably heard of sage oil, but more than likely this is the first time you're hearing anything about clary sage oil. Well, you can consider this to be the cousin of regular sage oil. Although regular sage oil has similar benefits to clary sage oil, it has been shown to have more adverse reactions, and clary sage oil is the one that is preferred because it is much milder and safer.

The clary sage is a perennial herb that used to be found only in Syria, Italy, and Southern France. Nowadays, it is cultivated worldwide from European regions to Russia, from Morocco to the United States of America. This herb, called the Salvia Sclarea, grows from May to September. The clary sage oil is extracted from the leaves and buds of the clary sage herb by steam distillation.

Clary sage is used to treat eye health-related problems, it is an antidepressant, euphoric, anticonvulsant, antispasmodic, emmenagogue, and aphrodisiac, and it has other health benefits too.

COMMON USES OF CLARY SAGE OIL TODAY

Soothes eyes: Clary sage oil has been used for centuries to treat vision problems, such as strained or tired eyes. In fact, the word "clary" comes from the Latin word "clarus" which means clear, and it was frequently called "clear eyes" in the past. If you are having vision problems and want a natural product to improve your eyesight, then get some clary sage oil. Get some water and put a few drops of clary sage oil in it. Then soak a clean cloth in the mixture and press it over your eyes or the affected eye for at least ten minutes. Do this every day until your vision improves.

Antidepressant and Euphoric: Clary sage oil is the oil to use on days when you are feeling down. It has been shown to boost confidence, self-esteem, mental strength, and hope, and it is therefore very good at treating the different forms of depression. It induces feelings of pleasure and immense joy, and it will fill you with the desire to live your life to the fullest. Whether you are depressed because of loneliness, failures in your career or personal life, insecurity, death of a loved one, or any other reason, inhaling the diluted vapor of some clary sage oil can go a very long way in helping you feel better.

Anticonvulsant and Antispasmodic: Did you know that clary sage oil can be used in addition to the existing medications as a treatment for convulsions? Yes, it most definitely can! This is because clary sage oil reduces or calms down convulsions, whether they are caused by epilepsy or some other mental or nervous disorder. It relaxes the nerves and thereby prevents these convulsions from occurring. It is also good for treating spasms, spasmodic cholera, spasmodic coughs, respiratory system cramps, muscle cramps, stomachaches, and even headaches.

Emmenagogue: One of the widest-known uses of clary sage oil is for regulating the menses. Yes, that's right ladies – this all-natural product will regularize your periods, ease menstrual discomfort, and reduce the pain without any adverse side effects. There is no need to go to the gynecologist and spend a small fortune for him to prescribe you a drug which contains clary sage oil anyway; simply use the oil as a massage oil and rub it into your lower abdomen and into your lower back if it hurts too.

Aphrodisiac: The men will smile when they read this other use of clary sage oil, and it is, in fact, true – clary sage oil is a potent aphrodisiac and has been used for ages to boost the libido. It increases the testosterone levels in both men and women, and this leads to increases in sexual interest and performance. So if you feel that you have fallen off the horse in that area and you want to get back up, use three drops of the clary sage oil and massage it into your hands and face.

Clary sage oil is safe for ingestion and has been used in the past to fight bacteria that live in the digestive system. It exhibits moderate antibacterial activity against various bacterial strains, such as Klebsiella, Staphylococcus aureus, Proteus mirabilisspecies, and Listeria monocytogenes. It is also very good at killing dangerous fungal strains such as the Penicillium, Aspergillus, Fusarium, and the Candida species.

Women should avoid clary sage oil during pregnancy because it stimulates menstrual flow. It should also be kept away from women who need to regulate their estrogen levels.

GERANIUM OIL

The geranium plant is a perennial shrub with pointy leaves and small pink flowers that is indigenous to South Africa. There are many varieties of this shrub, but the Pelargonium graveolens is the variety used to make the renowned geranium essential oil. Like the lavender and clary sage oils, the geranium essential oil is extracted from the leaves and stalks of the plant via steam distillation.

The geranium oil is mostly used today to stop hemorrhaging, promote cell health, and increase urination, among other things.

COMMON USES OF GERANIUM OIL TODAY

Hemostatic: I bet you wouldn't believe me if I told you that geranium can be used to stop hemorrhaging, or bleeding as the layman would call it. Geranium stops hemorrhaging in two different ways. Firstly, it causes the blood vessels to contract, so it restricts and eventually stops the flow of blood from damaged arteries, veins, and capillaries. Secondly, it speeds up blood clotting and thereby aids in the healing of wounds. By stopping excessive hemorrhaging, geranium helps to prevent toxins from entering your wounds and thereby causing an infection. Dilute the geranium and place it over your cuts and bruises to stop the excessive bleeding.

Cytophylactic: In addition to being a hemostatic, geranium also helps your body by promoting cell health, encouraging the regeneration of new cells and the recycling of dead cells. This helps all body cells, including the gametes, and improves the body's metabolism.

Diuretic: Geranium increases urination. After reading this, I'm sure many of you are smiling; "Why would I want to increase my urination?" you may ask. Well, urination is one of three methods that the body uses to rid itself of toxins. The other methods are perspiration and excretion, but urination is arguably the most important of them all. When you urinate, you are eliminating toxins such as uric acid, urea, bile salts, pathogens, heavy metals, some pollutants, harmful synthetic and chemical substances, and sometimes even excess sugar. The more you urinate, the lower your blood pressure will be because each time you urinate, you eliminate sodium, and this helps to reduce blood pressure. So, you see, by increasing your urination frequency, geranium helps to make you healthier and toxin-free.

Deodorant: The uplifting and pleasing aroma of geranium oil is all you'll need to keep those areas smelling wonderfully. It is mild on the skin, it has a long-lasting smell, and its antibacterial properties will keep you smelling fresh for a long time. So put some geranium on a clean washcloth and rub it on those areas that you need to keep fresh throughout the day.

Vermifuge: For those of you reading who suffer from intestinal worms, geranium essential oil is the oil for you! Geranium will kill all of your pesky internal parasitic worms, and it can even be used in children too. Drink three to five drops of geranium per day and those pesky parasites shall be no more.

Neural Degeneration: One of the saddest parts of aging is the neural generation that sometimes takes place and the dependency that comes with it. Wouldn't you like to protect yourself and the ones you love from neurodegenerative diseases such as dementia and Alzheimer's? If your answer is yes, then you need to be using geranium essential oil. It has been proven to activate microglial cells, cells which are integral components in the fight against neural degeneration. When microglial cells are activated, they reduce pro-inflammatory substances like nitric oxide, which fights off inflammation that cause neural degeneration in the neural pathways. Geranium oil has a synergistic relationship with the brain, and if you use it on a regular basis, you can prevent those dangerous and potentially deadly neural degenerative diseases. Place a few drops of geranium in your food every day and you will be well on your way to fighting off neural degeneration.

Astringent: An astringent is a substance used to shrink or constrict body tissues. Geranium oil tends to function as an astringent in that it makes the muscles, gums, skins, intestines, blood, and tissues contract. This includes the muscles of the abdomen, which gives you toned look. It also prevents the skin from sagging and helps prevent tooth loss by tightening up the gums, and it is very good at reducing wrinkles because it tightens facial skin. So if you want to look younger, fresher, and more toned, add three to four drops of geranium oil in your body lotion and apply it to your skin daily.

Geranium can also be used in the treatment of dermatitis, acne, eczema, and other skin ailments as well as infections of the throat, nose, and other respiratory organs. Geranium is good for treating ulcers, burns, neuralgia, tonsillitis, and also Post Menopausal Syndrome (PMS). It is great for improving both mental functioning and moods and is therefore widely used in the treatment of chronic anxiety and depression, and it is sometimes used in anger management.

Geranium is commonly blended with bergamot, angelica, lavandin, lavender, basil, carrot seed, cedar wood, citronella, jasmine, lemon, orange, lime, grapefruit, and rosemary oil.

Geranium is not recommended for use in pregnant women or in women who are breast-feeding. It should also not be used on babies or young children.

SANDALWOOD OIL

Sandalwood oil has been used in the religious festivals and shrines of India since prehistoric times. It is an expensive oil, and the demand for it is very high, but the numbers of trees available to make it are dwindling by the second. The sandalwood tree, Santalum album, is parasitic and very difficult to propagate; in fact, the tree must grow for at least thirty years before it is suitable for harvesting. When the tree is harvested at this time, it contains a significant amount of heartwood, the most precious part of the sandalwood tree. Nowadays, the sandalwood oil is extracted mainly by steam distillation, but back in the day, hydro-distillation was the primary method used to extract it. It is said that the hydro-distillation method yields an oil which has a very fine aroma.

It is best known in the western world as a rich, warm, sweet, and woody essential oil used as an ingredient in fragrant products, such as perfumes, cosmetics, and aftershaves. It has many benefits; it is an antiseptic, an anti-inflammatory, and a "cicatrisant" among other things.

Antiseptic: Sandalwood oil acts as a very good antiseptic agent. What is interesting to note about this antiseptic is that it is safe for both internal and external use and can help to protect internal ulcers and wounds from infection. It performs the same job when it is applied topically – it protects sores, wounds, pimples, and boils from becoming septic. So the next time you find yourself with a sore, don't be afraid to use a few drops of sandal wood oil on the sore to protect it from microbes.

Anti-inflammatory: The essential oil of sandalwood and also its paste are very good at providing relief from many different types of inflammation, including inflammations of the digestive, excretory, circulatory, and nervous systems. It is especially useful in cases of circulatory and nervous inflammations and can be used to get the affected organ system back up and running in no time. Simply place three to four drops of the sandalwood oil in a glass of water to begin with and increase the concentration if the mixture is not potent enough. Drink this every day until your condition ameliorates.

Cicatrisant: Sandalwood oil is great for soothing the skins of both young children and adults. In fact, it not only soothes the skin, but it also helps scars and abrasions heal much quicker. It can be placed in lotions, oils, etc. and moisturized into the skin for positive results. The potent healing effects of sandalwood oil have now sparked many producers of skin care creams, lotions, and soaps to include the oil as part of their main ingredients. So the next time you take up your beauty lotion, check out the label and see if you have already been reaping some benefits of sandalwood oil.

Carminative: Sandalwood oil induces relaxation wherever it is applied, even in the intestines. As such, when it is ingested, it relaxes the abdominal and intestinal muscles and makes it much easier for the excess gases there to escape. It also helps to prevent the formation of excess gases in the first place, and this is great because we all know how embarrassing it can be when those gases escape at the wrong place and time. A few drops of sandalwood in your water is all the carminative you will ever need.

Expectorant: An expectorant is a substance that loosens congestion in your chest, thereby making it easier for you to cough. Sandalwood oil works miracles in this area and has been used for a long time as an expectorant to treat blocked-up bronchioles and lungs. Simply massage a few drops of the oil into your chest and throat and all the phlegm that has been preventing you from breathing properly will come out in the blink of an eye.

Hypotensive: Just when you thought that sandalwood essential oil could not get any better, it just did! Another great quality of sandalwood oil is that it can be used to lower blood pressure. This means that it should be in the house of every person suffering from hypertension. It may be ingested for this purpose or it can also be applied topically – it would still have the same effect of lowering the blood pressure in that localized area.

Memory Booster: Sandalwood stimulates your mind, improves your memory, and increases your power of concentration. It is especially good for students because it does all of this and also relieves stress and anxiety. Students are especially prone to stress and tension, and sandalwood oil will work wonders in their lives and help them to perform at their very best.

Tonic: Sandalwood oil is soothing on the stomach and on the nervous, circulatory, and digestive systems. Therefore, it can be used by children of all ages, and it is a very good health tonic for everyone.

BERGAMOT OIL

The nearly ripe fruit of the bergamot orange tree, Citrus bergamia, is cold-pressed or hand-pressed to yield the bergamot essential oil. This tree was made by crossbreeding an orange tree and a lemon tree, and the fruit is yellow with a pear-like shape. About one hundred bergamot oranges will produce only eighty-five grams, or three ounces, of the bergamot oil. Although it had its origins in South East Asia, it was more widely produced in the coastal, southern section of Italy, such as in Sicily and Reggio di Calabria. In fact, the fruit was named after the city of Bergamo found in Lombardy, Italy, where it was commonly sold. The bergamot orange tree is also grown in Brazil, Turkey, Morocco, Argentina, and the Ivory Coast.

Bergamot has been used for ages for a variety of purposes; some of the most important uses are discussed below.

COMMON USES OF BERGAMOT OIL TODAY

Used in cosmetics, deodorants, fresheners: Bergamot oil has a unique aroma that is subtly spicy yet uniquely fruity. As such, the oil is frequently added to cosmetic products, perfumes, sprays, and many air fresheners. In fact, bergamot oil is a major component of the original 4711 Eau De Cologne made by Johann Maria Farina in Germany at the beginning of the eighteenth century. Bergamot oil is also used as a deodorant because of its fresh aroma and its disinfectant properties. It inhibits the growth of odor-causing germs, and its strong citrus smell is very pleasing to the nose. To use bergamot oil as a deodorant, simply dampen a clean washcloth with it and apply it to your underarms.

Fruity flavoring: Bergamot is used for its distinct flavoring in popular teas such as Lady Grey and Earl Grey. It is also used in Norway in the bergamot-flavored snus, a sugar-free, smokeless tobacco from the eighteenth century. In Turkey, many confectionaries are flavored with bergamot.

Stimulant, antidepressant, and relaxant: Bergamot oil has certain substances, such as limonene and alpha pinene, that are natural stimulats and antidepressants.

They create a feeling of joy, freshness, and energy in cases of depression and sadness by improving the circulation of blood. They also help to maintain proper metabolic rates by stimulating hormonal secretions. This stimulating effect increases the secretion of insulin, bile, and digestive juices, thereby helping the digestive and assimilative processes in the body. It aids in the decomposition of sugars and thereby lowers blood sugars because of this property. Add a few drops of bergamot oil to your vaporizer and inhale the sweet aroma; you will feel happier and stronger too.

Bergamot oil also contains many different flavonoids that act as relaxants too. They will soothe your nerves and reduce your stress, anxiety, and tension. This can help to cure or treat illnesses such as depression, insomnia, high blood pressure, and sleeplessness. In addition, bergamot oil stimulates the activity of certain hormones like serotonin and dopamine that induce feelings of sedation and relaxation.

Analgesic: If you are tired of taking heavy dosages of analgesic pills for muscle aches, sprains, terrible headaches, and other ailments, then you can substitute bergamot oil in place of them. By doing this, you also avoid the dangerous side effects of those over-the-counter medicines too. Bergamot essential oil reduces feelings of pain in your body by stimulating the secretion of hormones that lessen the sensitivity of your nerves to pain. Rub an ample amount of the bergamot oil into the affected area and the pain that you are feeling there will quickly subside.

Digestive: Do you want to improve your digestive system and prevent gastrointestinal complications too? If your answer is yes, then bergamot oil can come to your rescue. It increases the secretions of digestive acids and enzymes and activates them also. It increases the secretion of bile, facilitates easier digestion by regulating peristaltic motion of the intestines, and reduces strains on the intestinal tract. It therefore regularizes bowel movements, reduces constipation, and effectively prevents gastrointestinal complications such as colorectal cancer and other dangerous conditions. Give your digestive system a boost by drinking three to four drops of bergamot in some milk or honey every day.

Febrifuge: A febrifuge is a substance that lowers bodily temperature and thereby reduces fevers. Bergamot acts as an excellent febrifuge for numerous reasons. Firstly, it has antibiotic and other anti-microbial properties that help to fight off infections from the protozoa, viruses, and bacteria that usually cause fevers. That includes the malaria protozoa, the influenza virus, and the typhoid bacteria. Secondly, bergamot oil stimulates glandular secretions and also boosts the metabolic system. Both these actions will help to reduce toxicity in the body, clean out the glands, and help fight off the fever. To use bergamot oil as a febrifuge, simply use it to massage the whole body, especially the head and neck. You should also encourage the person with the fever to breathe in the relaxing aroma.

Cicatrisant: Being a cicatrisant, bergamot oil will help your scars and other marks disappear by evenly distributing the pigments in the skin to which it is applied. This will result in marks fading over time and revealing attractive, evenly-toned skin. This oil can be especially useful for those who suffer from terrible acne that can leave noticeable marks and scars on the skin for years. The ability of bergamot oil to act as a cicatrisant has caused many skin care product manufacturers and cosmetic manufacturers to use it in their creams, beauty soaps, and lotions. You can place a few drops of the bergamot in your lotion and beauty cream, or you can add it to a clean washcloth and apply it to the affected areas directly.

It is important to note that one of the main components of bergamot essential oil is bergaptene, a substance that becomes poisonous when it is exposed to sunlight. As such, bergamot essential oil must always be protected from sunlight, and it should always be stored in dark areas and in dark bottles. You should try to avoid direct sunlight exposure for at least forty-eight hours after applying bergamot essential oil to your skin.

Bergamot essential oil blends well with cedarwood, clary sage, ho leaf, geranium, neroli, citronella, lavender, frankincense, jasmine, mandarin, palmarosa, lemon, tangerine, rosewood, cypress, black pepper, geranium, rosemary, orange, sandalwood, nutmeg, betiver, and Ylang-ylang oil.

YLANG-YLANG OIL

The soft, sweet, flowery fragrance of the ylang-ylang oil has made it a romantic favorite around the world. It is steam distilled from the flowers of the ylang-ylang tree, the Cananga odorata, and the name ylang-ylang literally means flower of flower. In Indonesia, the flowers of the ylang-ylang tree are strewn across the beds of recently married couples.

The quality of ylang-ylang essential oil that is obtained from the ylang-ylang plant depends very much on the time of day that the flowers are picked. Early morning is the best time to pick the flowers because at this time the highest quantity and also the best quality of oil is available.

Antidepressant: If you are feeling down and you do not want to try any of the other essential oils above for your bad mood, why not try ylang-ylang? ylang-ylang has been used as a powerful antidepressant for years, and it fights depression by relaxing the mind and body. It induces feelings of hope and joy and thereby fights off those negative feelings of sadness, anxiety, or chronic stress which may be getting you down. Even those who are undergoing a nervous breakdown or some acute shock can benefit from the Ylang-Ylang essential oil.

Antiseborrhoeic: Seborrhoeic eczema, or seborrhea for short, is a distressing disease that occurs when our sebaceous glands malfunction. It causes the irregular production of sebum and the consequent infection of the cells of the epidermis. It is very painful and unattractive and results in pale yellow or white skin that easily peels off. This peeling usually takes place on the eyebrows, cheeks, scalp, and wherever else hair follicles are found. Ylang-ylang essential oil has been the leader in curing the inflammatory situation that seborrhoeic eczema brings; it reduces skin irritation and redness by treating the infection while regularizing sebum production. Start by applying six drops of ylang-ylang oil to a clean wash cloth and apply it to the skin two times daily; you may increase the concentration if needed.

Antiseptic: With every wound that you or your family gets, there comes with it the chance of a serious infection from bacteria and other microorganisms. The risk of complications is even higher when the wound was made by an iron object, as there remains a chance of it becoming infected by tetanus-causing germs. Protect yourself and your family by treating your wounds with ylang-ylang oil which protects the wounds from viruses, bacteria, and fungi and hence tetanus or sepsis. It also helps to speed up the healing process of the wound.

Aphrodisiac: If you want to reactivate or improve the romance between you and your sweetie, ylang-ylang can really help to give you that boost. It is very beneficial for those who have lost interest in sex due to depression, stress, or tremendous work load. Sometimes, due to the stress of modern life, we may lose our libido, but that should not be considered a permanent situation. Rub ylang-ylang essential oil all over your body when you need that extra drive.

Hypotensive: High blood pressure has been a growing problem for both the young and old in recent years. In addition, the hypotensive drugs being used to lower blood pressure have been having adverse effects on the health of those who use them. Ylang-ylang oil is a natural and effective alternative that can be used to lower blood pressure in the hypertensive.

Nervine: Ylang-ylang essential oil is very effective at boosting the nervous system. It repairs any damages to the nervous system and strengthens it. It protects the nerves from numerous different disorders and reduces stress on the nerves as well. Place a few drops of the ylang-ylang essential oil in your drinks daily and give your nervous system a healthy boost.

Ylang-ylang essential oil has also been used to cure infections of some internal organs including the intestines, stomach, urinary tract, and colon. It helps those who suffer from fatigue, insomnia, frigidity, and other stress-related conditions. It is very effective at keeping the skin looking young and supple, and it helps to keep it hydrated by maintaining the oil and moisture balance in the skin.

Some cases of headache, nausea, and sensitivity have been observed when people take the ylang-ylang essential oil in excessive amounts. When it is taken in the recommended doses, it is non-toxic and does not cause any irritation.

Ylang-ylang oil blends well with other essential oils such as sandalwood, lavender, grapefruit, and bergamot.

CHAPTER 7
ESSENTIAL OILS FOR BEAUTY

As you can see, most essential oils are multitalented and can help you improve a number of different aspects of your life. Yet there are some essential oils that are adapted specifically for improving beauty. Whether it is improving the quality of hair, nails, or skin, these essential oils will have you looking radiant and at your best when you use them as recommended.

ROSE AND ITS MANY DERIVATIVES

Most people associate roses with romance and their sweet smells, but did you know that rose oils can work wonders on your skin? Extracts of the delicate rose flower may be used on all skin types, and they are commonly included in skin care products for mature, sensitive, or dry skin.

The two rose species that are generally used in skin care are the Rosa centifola and the Rosa damascena. The Rosa damascena hails from Bulgaria and has a deep and potent smell; the Rosa centifola, known by some as the Moroccan rose or the cabbage rose, has a clean, light, and sweet smell. Both are valued for the essential oils that come from their flowers, and it takes tens of thousands of rose blossoms to make 1 ounce of rose essential oil. This makes rose oil one of the most expensive essential oils around, but the good thing is that the unadulterated oil is very concentrated, and so a few drops can go a long way. The blossoms are picked as they are unfolding in the wee hours of dawn.

Rose oil contains an intricate array of antioxidants, minerals, and vitamins that make it an excellent emollient for moisturizing dull and dry skin. It also has astringent, antiseptic, and anti-inflammatory properties to tighten the skin, treat acne, and reduce inflammation and redness. Rose oil is often used in the control of skin diseases such as atopic dermatitis and psoriasis, and it is great at refining skin texture. A study recently conducted on rose oil has even proven that it helps in the healing of wounds of the skin, and when you inhale it, it lowers the concentration of the stress hormone cortisol in your body and decreases the amount of water that is lost from your skin. Rub a few drops of the rose oil into the skin of the affected area and relax while it heals it from the inside out.

In addition to all the properties described above, rose essential oil also helps you look more beautiful by calming and soothing you. The happier you are, the more beautiful you will look, and rose oil can go a long way in making you feel happier and more energized. Add a few drops of the rose essential oil to your bath water daily and you will see the difference in the quality and texture of your skin.

Another derivative from the rose plant is the rosehip seed oil. This time, it is taken from the small fruits that sit behind the flowers of the Rosa moschata or Rosa rubigniosa. Rosehip seed oil is rich in proteins and oils, and it contains high levels of vitamin C. All these properties help to keep your skin soft and moisturized. It is also the only vegetable oil around that naturally contains vitamin A/retinol. Retinol is extremely useful in the treatment of wrinkles, lines and other signs of aging on the skin. Rosehip oil also slows down the formation of pigments, such as sun spots or age spots, so it is a common ingredient in the popular brands of anti-aging creams, skin lighteners, and sunscreens. You can safely add the rosehip oil to your favorite lotions and creams; it will only help to enhance their moisturizing and protective effects.

The final essential oil that is derived from roses that we will talk about in this book is rosewater or rose hydrosol; some people may know it as rose distillate or rose floral water. To obtain the rose hydrosol, the small patches of rose buds are steamed in copper distilleries to release the volatile therapeutic compound into the water. It is an intricate process, and the essential oil is drawn off and the rose hydrosol, which contains constituents of the flower and the micro-molecules of the essential oil, is captured drop by drop. It is often used in hair tonics, toners, and facial mists because its antibacterial properties help to protect and also balance the skin. Put some rosewater in your shampoo when you wash your hair or use it as your personal hair oil. Your hair and scalp will thank you for it.

JASMINE

Jasmine is one of the most famous flowers you will ever come across. No matter where you go in the world, there is always someone who will be familiar with its pleasing yet sweet and romantic fragrance. The flowers are beautiful and they only bloom at night, filling the air with their alluring fragrance. The word Jasmine is Persian in origin and is derived from the word that means "a gift from God." The name Jasmine is a common name for girls in the Indian subcontinent and also in the Middle Eastern region. The flower is associated with love and romance and has been the inspiration for many poets since the dawn of time.

The jasmine essential oil is extracted from the flowers of the jasmine plant by steam distillation. The variety of jasmine that is mainly used is the jasminum officinale. The jasminum grandiflora is also commonly used.

Jasmine has long been used for skin care and for treating dehydrated, brittle, and dry skin. It may cause an allergic reaction if it is used on open wounds or cracked skin, so care must be taken. Nonetheless, it is still used in the treatment of dermatitis and eczema and is very effective in curing these ailments. Simply rub a few drops of the oil into the affected areas daily before going to bed.

Jasmine also helps to restore skin elasticity. It is good for fading scars and stretch marks, and it helps to evenly tone all different types of skin, from sensitive to irritated to dry to greasy.

ARGAN OIL

Its alias alone lets you know what a treasure this essential oil is: argan oil, also known as liquid gold. It is derived from the gigantic argan tree, Argania spinosa, which can grow to be several meters tall and is native to Morocco. The argan oil itself is derived from the kernels of the argan tree, and it is extremely rich in nutrients such as vitamin E and fatty acids. It is this abundance of beneficial nutrients, which make it great for the skin and hair, and it is a popular oil of choice for many celebrities who can afford to buy it in abundance. This oil is not only for the rich and famous; anyone can use argan oil to affect positive changes in their body.

Argan oil is very hydrating, and as such, it is commonly used as a skin moisturizer to soften the skin. It is absorbed into the skin easily, and it is non-irritating as well as non-oily. It can be used all over the body, including the neck and face. Simply smooth a few drops of the oil into your skin after cleansing and gently rub it in as you would any other body or face lotion. You can use it as a serum by applying your night cream after the oil has been absorbed into your skin. You can also place a few drops of the Argan oil into your bath water or body lotion and you will still reap the same positive results. It is safe for use even on a baby's tender skin.

You can use brown sugar, vanilla extract, and argan oil to create an exquisite exfoliating lip scrub and moisturizer. Just add a few drops of the argan oil to some fine brown sugar and vanilla extract (enough to cover your lips). Massage it lightly into your lips using a circular motion and then rinse it off for sexier lips.

If you are tired of your old facemask or if you want to give it an organic lift, just add some argan oil to the mix. Three drops of argan oil, a tablespoon of honey, three teaspoons of Greek-style yogurt, and a tablespoon of lemon juice will be the best homemade rejuvenating and brightening facemask you will ever need. Apply it to a clean, dry face, and leave it on for at least ten minutes. Then wash it off with some warm water. If you cannot take the hassle of making your own facemask, simply mix in a few drops of the argan oil into your store-bought mask for extra skin rejuvenation.

People who suffer from eczema often have itchy, flaky, and raw skin and even they can benefit immensely from the repairing power of argan oil. The fatty acid and vitamin E content provide the skin with the nutrients it needs to repair itself, and it will also prevent further damage and irritation. To reduce eczema, apply a small amount of the argan oil directly on the affected skin and massage it gently into the skin until all of it has been absorbed. Other types of skin that are sore, cracked, irritated, or damaged can also benefit from a daily dosage of argan oil. It will sooth the pain and reduce the inflammation, and, as said before, it will increase the rate of healing. Even stretch marks can be minimized by the daily application of argan oil to the area.

Acne is another skin condition that agonizes many across the world. Are you tired and fed up of using those store-bought moisturizers and oils that only exacerbate your acneic condition? If your answer is yes, then choose argan oil all the way! It is non-greasy and will help to balance your skin by providing natural moisture. It is also filled with natural antioxidants that help to reduce inflammation and heal damaged skin cells.

Apply a few drops of your argan oil to your acne-afflicted skin after you clean it and pat it dry. Rub it gently into your skin two times daily for mild acne, or you may even make more applications for chronic acne. Then simply relax and kiss your acne woes goodbye forever.

If you find yourself with tough heels and cuticles, it is time you pick up a bottle of argan oil. Massage a few drops of the oil into your cuticles daily to soften them and encourage nail growth. You can use the argan oil as an overnight treatment for your cracked or damaged heels. Simply massage an ample amount into your feet and toes before you go to bed. Cover them with a sock and you will wake up to healthier and softer feet.

If you thought argan oil was only good for your skin and nails, then you thought wrong. It can also work miracles for your hair and scalp too! Argan oil has also been proven to make hair shinier, silkier, and softer; it is the perfect conditioner as it moisturizes and protects hair, conditions hair, and makes it silky smooth. It helps to treat split ends and it tames frizzy hair too. What more could you ask for in a conditioner? Substitute it in place of your useless store-bought conditioner the next time you wash your hair and you will be pleasantly surprised by the results.

CHAPTER 8
AROMATHERAPY

Aromatherapy is the science and art of using naturally extracted essential oils from plants to harmonize, balance, and promote the health of spirit, mind, and body. It aims to unify spiritual, psychological, and physiological processes to enhance an individual's innate healing process. Simply put, aromatherapy is using the aroma of essential oils to heal the mind, body, and soul.

You can rub the diluted oils into your skin and breathe in the pleasing aroma. You can add a few drops of the essential oils to water in a spray bottle and use it as an air freshener, or you can make a scented candle by placing one or two drops of the oil in the melted wax of the lit candle. Can you think of any other ways in which you can enjoy the pleasing aroma of essential oils? While you do that, let me introduce you to some other essential oils that are great for aromatherapy.

LEMON ESSENTIAL OIL

Lemon oil is a favorite because of its therapeutic qualities and clean scent. It eases the symptoms of arthritis and acne, and it aids in digestion and concentration. It comes from the citrus limonum plant, and the oil is extracted from the peel via cold expression. Add a few drops of the lemon oil to your diffuser or vaporizer to enhance your energy. Or add it to your lotion, massage it into your skin, and inhale the pleasing aroma. For an immune system boost, add a few drops to your bath water and let it soak into your skin while you inhale the aroma.

Do not use lemon oil if you plan to go out into the sun because certain compounds within it may react with the UV rays from the sun to create harmful substances.

TEA TREE ESSENTIAL OIL

The tea tree essential oil is extracted from the stems and leaves of the Melaleuca alternifolia plant via steam distillation. You can add it to your diffuser or vaporizer and inhale it and be revitalized, or you can apply it to your skin in many different ways. Mix the tea tree essential oil with your favorite cream, oil, or lotion and massage it into your skin or add it to your bath water. You can also massage a few drops of the tea tree essential oil directly into your skin for an instant uplift. Tea tree essential oil is a known immune system booster and it helps to fight off infections.

PEPPERMINT ESSENTIAL OIL

Put the pep back in your step by whiffing some peppermint essential oil today. It is a perennial herb that is known to boost energy, enhance mental alertness, and have a refreshing, cool effect. Peppermint essential oil is extracted via steam distillation from the mentha piperita, and it is commonly found in mouthwash, baths, lotions, massage oil, and vaporizers. It also enhances moods, combats irritation and redness, aids digestion, and alleviates symptoms of congestion.

Care must be taken when using peppermint, however, because the menthol it contains may be a bother to some people. Keep it away from small children and do not use it while you are pregnant.

ROSEMARY ESSENTIAL OIL

For a natural lift or memory boost, add a few drops of rosemary oil to your bath water or humidifier. Rosemary is a wonderful mental stimulant. It packs a powerful punch when it comes to aromatherapy and has been considered sacred for centuries.

The plant, Rosmarinus officinalis, is a woody, perennial herb, and the oil is extracted by steam distillation from the flowering part of the plant. It is known to relieve sinusitis and congestion issues and also enhance memory. You can blend it with your massage oils and lotions to help arthritis, aching, stiff muscles, gallbladder and liver congestion, and other digestive problems. You can also put it in your shampoo to make your hair grow and heal your scalp.

Rosemary should not be used by pregnant women, people with high blood pressure, or people with epilepsy.

EUCALYPTUS ESSENTIAL OIL

Eucalyptus oil has a powerful scent that is easily recognizable. It comes from the eucalyptus tree that is native to Australia. There are over five hundred varieties of eucalyptus trees, and the oil is steam distilled from the twigs and leaves of some. It has the ability to enhance concentration, and it is a very effective agent against respiratory diseases. Eucalyptus oil is also good for fighting off migraines and it too can be placed in a humidifier and inhaled.

Epileptics should avoid using eucalyptus oil. Women who are breast-feeding or pregnant should also avoid using the oil. If it is ingested in large doses, it can be fatal.

CHAPTER 9
COMMON AILMENTS AND THE ESSENTIAL OIL BLENDS THAT CAN BE USED TO CURE THEM

Maybe you do not want to make use of one single oil, but you want to mix them to whip up something that is especially formulated for a specific problem. Not to fear; essential oils will still come to the rescue.

SORE THROAT OR TONSILLITIS

Ingredients:
2 drops clove essential oil
3 drops geranium

Directions:
Mix in a diffuser and inhale deeply for sore throat relief. Alternatively, you can rub a drop of each of the ingredients listed above on your throat for the same sore throat relief.

CELLULITE

Ingredients:
20 drops grapefruit oil
20 drops geranium oil

Directions:
Mix the ingredients listed above into an ounce of sweet almond oil or fractionated coconut oil and apply it to the affected area daily

MOSQUITO REPELLENT

Ingredients:
1-2 drops lavender, rosemary, or tea tree oil
3-5 drops geranium

Directions:
Mix all the ingredients together well and apply it to the part of your skin that will be left exposed to the elements.

ACNE

Ingredients:
5 drops Manuka or New Zealand tea tree or regular tea tree essential oil
6 drops lavender essential oil
1 drop geranium essential oil
1 fluid ounce fractionated coconut oil or jojoba

Directions:

Pour the fractionated coconut oil or jojoba into a very clean bottle and then add the manuka, lavender, and geranium essential oils. Tightly close the bottle and roll it for a minute or two to mix the ingredients. Apply a small amount to your back, neck or face, but be certain to avoid the nostrils, the lips, the eyes, and inside the ears. Gently roll the bottle each time you use it to ensure that the essential oils are properly mixed

MENSTRUAL CRAMPS

Ingredients:
3 drops lavender essential oil
4 drops cypress essential oil
5 drops peppermint essential oil
1 fluid ounce jojoba

Directions:

Mix the lavender, cypress, and peppermint oils well with the jojoba. Mix them in a dark-colored, clean glass bottle and gently massage a small amount into your abdominal area whenever you are feeling cramps.

CONGESTION

Ingredients:
4 drops peppermint essential oil
25 drops ravensara essential oil

30 drops eucalyptus essential oil
Aromatherapy inhaler or cotton ball

Directions:
Mix the peppermint, ravensara, and eucalyptus oils in a dark-colored, clean glass bottle, preferably one with a built-in dropper insert or orifice reducer.

If you have the aromatherapy inhaler, soak the insert in the essential oil mixture that you created and insert it into the tube and secure the cap. Raise the inhaler to your nose and breathe in deeply as much as needed. You can also apply two to three drops to a cotton ball and inhale the essential oil mix from the cotton ball.

INSOMNIA

Ingredients:
5 drops bergamot essential oil
5 drops clary sage essential oil
10 drops roman chamomile essential oil

Directions:
Blend the bergamot, clary sage, and roman chamomile oils well in a dark-colored, clean glass bottle. Add one or two drops of the mixture you created in the step before to a tissue and place the tissue inside your pillow to help you fall asleep at night.

CONCLUSION

Essential oils are versatile gifts from nature that can be used to improve your life in many different ways. They are powerful substances that can help to heal your body, mind, and soul. There are different types of essential oils with each essential oil having its own unique set of benefits. They are one of the most potent all-round healers that nature has blessed us with, and, when combined, they can give an even stronger defense against common ailments and the occasional rare ones too. Some of them are quite volatile, but as long as you know how to use and store them safely, they will be with you for a very long time, and they will heal you from the inside out.

DID YOU LIKE "ESSENTIAL OILS FOR BEGINNERS"?

Before you go, I'd like to say "thank you so much" for purchasing my book.

I know you could have picked from dozens of books on this subject, but you took a chance with mine and I'm truly grateful for that.

So once again, a big thanks for downloading this book and reading all the way to the end, I truly appreciate it.

Now I'd like to ask for a small favor if you don't mind . . .

Would you be so kind as to take a minute of your time and leave a review for this book on Amazon.

This feedback will help me continue to write the kind of books that help you get results. And if you loved it then please feel free to let me know! :)